ZELLINGER-ELLISON SYNDROME

UNDERSTANDING EVERYTHING ABOUT
ZELLINGER-ELLISON SYNDROME

DR. AHMED .R

Contents

CHAPTER ONE

INTRODUCTION

A complex disorder known as Zollinger-Ellison syndrome occurs when a tumor forms in the duodenum, the upper portion of the small intestine, or the pancreas. The hormone gastrin, which is secreted in excess by these tumors known as gastrinomas, causes your stomach to create excessive levels of acid. Peptic ulcers are the result of too much acid.

Rare is the Zollinger-Ellison syndrome (ZES). Though the illness can strike at any stage of life, most cases are discovered in individuals between the ages of 30 and 50. The standard course of treatment for Zollinger-Ellison syndrome is taking medications that lower stomach acid and treat ulcers.

Symptoms

The following are possible Zollinger-Ellison syndrome signs and symptoms:

stomach ache

The diarrhea

Upper abdominal pain that feels burning, agonizing, gnawing, or uncomfortable

Heartburn and acid reflux

vomiting and nausea

Deficiency

bleeding within the digestive system

Unintentional loss of weight

Reduced desire to eat

Anemia

When to visit a physician

If you have a continuous upper abdominal ache that is burning, hurting, or gnawing, see your doctor. This is especially important if you have also been having nausea, vomiting, or diarrhea.

Inform your physician if you have taken over-the-counter acid-reducing drugs for an extended length of time, such as ranitidine (Zantac), omeprazole (Prilosec), cimetidine (Tagamet), or famotidine (Pepcid). Your symptoms might be concealed by these drugs, delaying your diagnosis. It's critical to have therapy and early detection if you have Zollinger-Ellison syndrome.

Reasons

It is still unclear what specifically causes Zollinger-Ellison syndrome. However, it is evident how the Zollinger-Ellison syndrome develops. The onset of the illness is attributed to the formation of a tumor (gastrinoma) in one or more of the duodenum, pancreatic, or surrounding lymph nodes.

Located beneath and behind your stomach is your pancreas. It generates the enzymes needed for food digestion. In addition, the pancreas generates a number of hormones, one of which is gastrin, which regulates the formation of stomach acid. In the duodenum, the section of the small intestine that is next to your stomach, digestive juices from the pancreas, liver, and gallbladder combine. This is the point at which digestion peaks.

The cells that make up the tumors associated with Zollinger-Ellison syndrome secrete a lot of gastrin, which causes the stomach to create an excessive amount of acid. The overabundance of acid subsequently causes diarrhea and occasionally peptic ulcers.

In addition to producing too much acid, the tumors could be malignant (cancerous). Although the tumors themselves develop slowly, the cancer can spread to other areas of your body, most commonly to your liver or neighboring lymph nodes.

Connection to Men I

Multiple endocrine neoplasia, type I (MEN I) is a hereditary disorder that may be the cause of Zollinger-Ellison syndrome. In addition to pancreatic tumors, people with MEN I also have several endocrine system tumors. In addition, they may have pituitary tumors as well as parathyroid gland tumors. About 25% of patients with gastrinomas have MEN I gastrinomas.

Getting Ready for Your Consultation

Even though your symptoms could make you see a general practitioner or your family doctor, a gastroenterologist a medical professional who specializes in disorders of the digestive system will probably be recommended to you in order to diagnose and treat Zollinger-Ellison syndrome. An oncologist a medical professional who specializes in treating cancer may also be recommended to you.

Here are some tips to help you prepare for your visit and understand what to anticipate from your physician.

CHAPTER TWO

What you're capable of

Read any restrictions about appointments in advance. Tell the staff of your doctor when you schedule the appointment whether you take any drugs. Proton pump inhibitors are among the medications that reduce acidity and may change the outcomes of certain tests used to diagnose Zollinger-Ellison syndrome. But don't stop taking these drugs without first talking to your doctor.

Jot down any symptoms you're having, even if they don't appear connected.

Important personal details, such as significant stressors or recent life transitions, should be included. Note down any medical history your family may have had as well.

Enumerate all the drugs, vitamins, and supplements you are currently taking.

Prepare a list of inquiries for your physician.

Questions to put to your physician

Basic inquiries for Zollinger-Ellison syndrome include the following:

What is probably the root of my illness or symptoms?

Do my symptoms have any other probable explanations besides Zollinger-Ellison syndrome?

Which tests are necessary to verify the diagnosis? How do I get ready for those exams?

What is the Zollinger-Ellison syndrome typical course of treatment?

Exist any other choices?

Which course of action would you suggest taking?

Do I have to adhere to any dietary restrictions?

Should I consult a specialist?

Is the medication you're giving for me available in generic form?

Which websites would you suggest reading up on to find out more about Zollinger-Ellison syndrome?

Does the fact that I have Zollinger-Ellison syndrome increase my risk of developing any other medical conditions?

How frequently must I return for follow-up appointments?

Which way do I stand?

What to anticipate from your physician

You will probably be asked a lot of questions by your doctor, such as:

When did you start feeling the effects?

Do you experience constant symptoms, or do they come and go?

What level of severity do you have?

What helps alleviate your problems, if anything?

What makes your symptoms worse, if anything?

Have you ever received a diagnosis of stomach ulcers? How was the diagnosis made?

Have you or any family members received a type I diagnosis of multiple endocrine neoplasia?

Have you or anybody in your family received a diagnosis of thyroid, pituitary, or parathyroid issues?

Has someone ever told you that your blood calcium level is high?

Your physician's diagnosis will be based on the following:

medical background. In addition to reviewing your medical history, your doctor will inquire about your symptoms and indicators. You have a higher chance of having Zollinger-Ellison syndrome if you have a blood relative with MEN I, such as a sibling or parent.

blood examinations. To determine if your levels of gastrin are elevated, a sample of your blood is examined. Elevated gastrin can be caused by a number of different illnesses, but it can also be an indication of pancreatic or duodenal cancers. To obtain the best accurate measurement of your gastrin levels, you may need to cease taking any medications that reduce acid and fast before the test. This test might be conducted multiple times due to the variability of gastrin levels.

measurement of the gastrin level. Your doctor may test the acidity of your stomach to determine which condition is causing your elevated gastrin levels, as conditions other than Zollinger-Ellison can also cause excessive gastrin levels. Additionally, if you take acid-blocking drugs or if your stomach doesn't produce any acid, your levels of glutathione may also be raised. Your doctor could administer a secretin stimulation test to see whether your stomach is producing acid. Your doctor will measure your gastrin levels for this test, inject you with the hormone secretin, and then recheck your gastrin levels. Your gastrin levels will rise even further if you have Zollinger-Ellison syndrome.

upper digestive tract endoscopy. Your doctor will sedate you and then use an endoscope a small, flexible device with a light and video camera to look for ulcers by passing it down your throat, into your stomach, and into your duodenum. Your doctor may take a biopsy (a sample of tissue removed from your duodenum) using an endoscope in order to examine it and look for tumors that produce gastrin. Your doctor will advise you to avoid eating anything after midnight the night before the test in order to prepare for it.

imaging research. Your physician may employ imaging methods like CT, MRI, or nuclear scans, which use radioactive tracers to help find cancers.

ultrasound endoscopy. Using an endoscope equipped with an ultrasound probe, your doctor checks your duodenum and stomach during this operation. By enabling a more thorough examination of the digestive system, the probe facilitates the detection of malignancies. Using an endoscope, a tissue sample can also be extracted. The night before the test, you must fast until after midnight. You will also be sedated for the test.

To treat Zollinger-Ellison syndrome, physicians address both the ulcers and the tumors. Your doctor may not need to treat ulcers if they can remove the tumors.

Tumor treatment

Because the tumors in Zollinger-Ellison syndrome are frequently small and hard to find, removing them from the body requires a skillful surgeon. If you have a single tumor, your physician might be able to remove it surgically; however, if you have several tumors or tumors that have progressed to your liver, surgery might not be an option. On the other hand, your doctor might still advise removing a single, huge tumor if you have several.

Doctors sometimes suggest additional therapies to stop tumor growth, such as:

removing the majority of a liver tumor through debulking

attempting to kill the tumor by either employing heat to kill cancer cells (radiofrequency ablation) or by cutting off the blood supply (embolization)

administering medication intratumorally to alleviate symptoms of malignancy

Chemotherapy is used to attempt to slow tumor growth.

A transplant of the liver

These days, most acid production and ulcers are controlled with medicine, so more drastic surgical methods like cutting the nerves that produce acid secretion or removing the entire stomach are rarely used.

Handling too much acid

Almost always, excess acid production can be managed. Proton pump inhibitor medications are the initial course of treatment. The best drugs for lowering acid production in cases with Zollinger-Ellison syndrome are these ones. Strong medications known as proton pump inhibitors work by preventing the little "pumps" that are found inside acid-secreting cells from producing acid. Lansoprazole (Prevacid), omeprazole (Prilosec, Zegerid), pantoprazole (Protonix), rabeprazole (Aciphex), and esomeprazole (Nexium) are among the drugs that are frequently recommended. The Food and Drug Administration reports that long-term use of prescription proton pump inhibitors has been linked to an increased risk of hip, wrist, and spine fractures, particularly in those 50 years of age and older. The benefits of these drugs in inhibiting acid should be considered in relation to the minor risk involved.

In addition, your physician might recommend one of the following surgeries to cure peptic ulcers:

halt the bleeding of an ulcer

relieve an ulcer-related blockage

Seal the opening (perforation) that an ulcer has created in the duodenum or stomach wall.